TABLE OF CONTENT

INTRODUCTION

This eBook explains the dangers caused by using commercial products, ways to avert them and how to make products on your own using natural and kitchen ingredients which are skin and environment friendly. It also gives a step by step guide on how to do these skin products at the comfort of your home without the help of an expert. Make your skin chemical free by abstaining from products which gives less but are very expensive to afford, products which leads to the growth of diseases and death. Happy reading!!!

CHAPTER ONE

BODY CREAM AND LOTION

Body cream is a tenacious fluid made up of oil and fat emulsion with a healing aim used on the skin to achieve this aim.

Lotion is a low to medium viscid topical preparation applied to unbroken skin.

The both are forms of moisturizers or soothing agents that replenish loss moisture to the body. When selecting your body cream or lotion, you must watch out for creams with harsh chemicals, alcohol, acetic acids, benzophenone, coal tar e. t. c. when using body crème or lotion, it must not be used on the face as the face is more delicate and thinner part of the body which is more exposed to environmental factors than the body at large. Also, body crème or lotion causes clogged pores and acne because they are more creamier than the face crème and they contain more chemicals which are harmful to the face, that is why it is advisable to use homemade body crème or lotion which are more nutritious and friendly to the skin.

REASONS WHY WE USE BODY CREAM OR LOTION

1. It seals moisture into the skin whereby preventing it from drying.
2. Restore extra dry or rough skin to smooth and soft skin.
3. It makes the skin glow.
4. It helps remove dead skin and makes it supple.
5. It makes you to feel and smell good.

HOW TO MAKE BODY CREAM USING KITCHEN INGREDIENTS

1. SHEA BUTTER PACK
   Things needed are:
   - Vitamin E oil   1 tablespoon
   - Organic coconut oil   ¼ cup

-	Aloe vera gel	¾ cup
-	Beeswax	1 tablespoon
-	Shea butter	¼ cup
-	Essential oil	20 drops (optional)
-	Bentonite clay	1 tablespoon (optional)

Put beeswax, shea butter and coconut oil in a plate and place in a micro wave to melt, pour it into a blender or mixer and mix well, add vitamin E oil and essential oil (optional) and mix till it cools and slowly add the aloe vera and mix to form a smooth consistence, remove lotion and place in a small container with a lid. Your body lotion is ready for use.

2. GINGER MOISTENING CREAM
   Things needed are:

-	Cocoa butter	½ cup
-	Vitamin E oil	2 teaspoons
-	Apricot kernel oil	2 teaspoons
-	Light sesame oil	2 teaspoons
-	Ginger	2

Grate the ginger and extract the juice, put it in a plate, add all the ingredients and heat to melt or place it over a pot of boiling water, when it melts, add few drops of orange juice, mix well and pour into a jar and keep in a cool place.

3. STRAW BERRY CRÈME FOR OILY OR NORMAL SKIN
   Things needed are:

-	Apricot kernel oil	1 tablespoon
-	Sweet almond oil	1 ½ tablespoon
-	White beeswax	½ tablespoon
-	Strawberry juice or apricot	1 tablespoon
-	Benzoin	8 drops

Mash the strawberries or apricot and extract the juice, put the beeswax and all the other oils in a plate and place over a boiling water or micro wave to melt, when it melts, remove it from heat and add the juice quickly and mix the till a creamy or flossy consistence is seen, add the benzoin and mix till it is cool, pour into a jar and keep in a cool place.

4. BAKING SODA LOTION
   Things needed are:
   - Grated beeswax   2 tablespoons
   - Olive oil   ¼ cup
   - Coconut oil   ¼ cup
   - Baking soda   one eighth cup
   - Distilled water or rain water   ¼ cup

Dissolve the baking soda in water in a bowl, mix all the oils in a plate and place over boiling water to melt and hot, remove from heat and add the mixture of the baking soda slowly as you stir the oil mixture, stir briskly until the mixture thickens, pour into a jar and keep in a cool place.

5. VASELINE FOR SMOOTHER BODY AND FEET
   Things needed are:
   - Grated beeswax   one eighth cup
   - Olive oil   ½ cup

 Put the two ingredients in a sauce pan and let it melt over boiling water, remove from heat, stir and pour into a jar and keep at room temperature After soaking your feet and hands, dry it and apply this Vaseline before going to bed, after application, put on socks and hand gloves to retain the moisture.

6. ALMOND MOISTURIZER
   Things needed are:
   - Vitamin E capsules   3
   - Beeswax   ½ cup
   - Rose, sandal wood or lavender essential oil   10 drops

Put the almond oil or avocado oil in a sauce pan with beeswax and place over low heat to melt, when it melts, remove from heat, stir and add vitamin E capsules and essential oil to it and mix well, pour into a jar and store at room temperature. It can last for maximum of 30 days. This can be used for the face and body.

7. BODY BUTTER RECIPE

Things needed are:

- Shea butter   1 cup
- Almond oil   ½ cup
- Coconut oil   ½ cup

Melt shea butter and coconut oil over boiling water, add almond oil stir and add any essential oil of your choice and stir, place oil in a freezer or outside to chill and wait until oil as start to partially solidify then wipe until a butter like consistency is achieved and pour into a jar.

OR

Whip shea butter, almond oil and vitamin E in a low heat.

CHAPTER TWO

HOMEMADE HAIR CREAM

This is used to improve hair growth and softness. The things needed to do this hair cream are:

-	Rosemary essential oil	6 drops
-	Chamomile essential oil	5 drops
-	Bergamot	5 drops
-	Vitamin E oil	½ teaspoon
-	Sweet almond oil	¾ teaspoon
-	Jojoba oil	¾ teaspoon
-	Olive oil	½ tablespoon
-	Coconut oil	½ tablespoon
-	Shea butter	2 tablespoons

Melt the shea butter and coconut oil in a low heat for few seconds, add the remaining ingredients, stir well and pour into a container, refrigerate for some hours or overnight, remove and keep at room temperature, to be used within a month. Do not use too much to avoid hair looking greasy.

NON GREASY POMADE

The things needed for this pomade are:

-	Sandal wood essential oil	10 drops
-	Bentonite	2 teaspoons
-	Coconut oil	3 tablespoons
-	Beeswax	2 tablespoons

Melt beeswax by placing it over boiling water, as it melts, add coconut oil and stir, remove from heat and add bentonite clay and stir continuously as it cools then add the essential oil and pour into a jar to be kept for maximum of 3 weeks.

HOMEMADE HERBAL STYLING GEL

Things needed are as follows:

- Essential oil of your choice   6 drops
- Distilled water or filtered water   ½ cup
- Unflavored gelatin   ¼ teaspoon

Heat water and mix together with gelatin in a bowl, stir well and keep in the refrigerator for 3 hours. Once it is cool, add essential oil if desired and stir well, pour into a jar and store in the fridge. It should be refrigerated after use and to be kept for maximum of 2 weeks.

CHAPTER THREE

HOMEMADE HAIR SPRAY

All you need to do this product is to boil a cup of water, add one teaspoon of gelatin to it, and stir until the gelatin dissolves completely. Store in a spray bottle but needs to be place in hot water before use as it solidifies when cool; this recipe is safe for the body and the ozone layer.

OR

Chop one lemon into a bowl, add water and place over boiling water, simmer until mixture is reduced by half, drain water using a fine silk cloth and pour the liquid into a bottle that will fit a pump – type sprayer. Add ½ cup of water to thin the mixture if needed. This mixture should always be made fresh every few days and kept in the fridge between uses, it is good for children's hair as it includes no chemicals, and lemon can be substituted with orange in cases of dry hair.

NATURAL HAND SANITIZER

Things needed are:

- Vitamin E oil   ¼ teaspoon
- Aloe vera gel   8 tablespoons
- Witch hazel extract or high proof vodka   1 tablespoon
- Tea tree essential oil   30 drops
- Lavender essential oil   10 drops

Put all the essential oils and vitamin E oil into a bottle and shake well, add witch hazel oil or high proof vodka to the oils and shake well to mix, then add the aloe vera gel and shake vigorously. The presence of vitamin E and alcohol in this mixture will preserve it for several months, if you are not a fan of lavender oil, you can use any other anti bacterial oil of your choice. Shake the bottle well before each use.

CHAPTER FOUR

FACE WASH

1. ORANGE PACK

   Things needed are:
   - Liquid castile soap   8 tablespoons
   - Finely ground orange peel   1 teaspoon
   - Sweet orange essential oil   35 drops

Mix all these ingredients together and use to wash your face in the morning.

OR

   - Liquid castile soap   8 tablespoons
   - Grape fruit essential oil   5 drops
   - Lemon essential oil   15 drops
   - Lime essential oil   15 drops

Mix all these ingredients together and use to wash your face in the morning.

2. GERANIUM PACK

   Things needed are:
   - Liquid castile soap   8 tablespoons
   - Geranium essential oil   25 drops
   - Lavender essential oil   15 drops

Mix all ingredients together and use to wash your face in the morning.

3. TEA TREE PACK

   Things needed are:
   - Liquid castile soap   8 tablespoons
   - Eucalyptus essential oil   15 drops
   - Tea tree essential oil   25 drops

Mix all ingredients and use to wash the face in the morning.

4. PEPPERMINT PACK

   Things needed are:
   - Liquid castile soap   8 tablespoons
   - Peppermint essential oil   25 drops

Mix the two ingredients together and use to wash the face in the morning.

5. ROSEMARY PACK

   Things needed are:
   - Liquid castile soap   8 tablespoons
   - Basil essential oil   30 drops
   - Rosemary essential oil   10 drops

Mix all ingredients together and use to wash your face in the morning.

6. LEMON PACK

   Things needed are:
   - Liquid castile soap   8 tablespoons
   - Lavender essential oil   15 drops
   - Lemon essential oil   30 drops

Mix all ingredients together and use to wash your face in the morning.

NATURAL HOMEMADE BODY WASH

Things needed are:

- Vitamin E oil   1 teaspoon
- Honey   ¼ cup
- Liquid castile soap   ¼ cup
- Jojoba oil or sweet almond oil or olive oil or grape seed oil or sesame oil
  2 tablespoons
- Essential oil   60 drops

If your honey is creamy and thick, warm it to liquefy before use, if it is to be used for a baby less than six months old, essential oil should be omitted in the preparation and if children are to use in this body wash, then the essential oil should be reduced to half the required quantity.

Mix all ingredients together in a bottle with a squirt top and shake well, whenever you want to have your bath, just squirt mixture on your sponge or bath pouf and use to bath. Due to no addition of water to mixture during preparation, it is likely to stay fresh for a year.

CHAPTER FIVE

ESSENTIAL OIL AND THEIR USES

1. ROSEMARY ESSENTIAL OIL
   This oil is very good for acne, eczema and dermatitis, it is stimulates and restore your skin, but should not be used during pregnancy or breast feeding or those who are epileptic or suffering from high blood pressure.
2. GERANIUM ESSENTIAL OIL
   This oil is amazing on oily skin complexion, acne, eczema, dermatitis, mature skin and other problematic skin. As it cures these skin problems, it brightens and revitalizes dull skin.
3. LAVENDER ESSENTIAL OIL
   This oil is amazing for all skin types including sensitive skin as it is very gentle on the skin. It is also great on mature skin, acne, eczema, psoriasis and soothes itchy skin.
4. CHAMOMILE ESSENTIAL OIL
   This oil is amazing on dry and sensitive skin, eczema, acne and dermatitis.
5. PALMAROSAL ESSENTIAL OIL
   This oil moisturizes your skin, controls the production of oil in your skin and encourages the growth of new skin cells, very valuable in the production of any skin care products.
6. GRAPE SEED ESSENTIAL OIL
   This oil helps to tone your skin, an amazing cleansing agent for oily skin type and has no phototoxic element.
7. PEPPERMINT ESSENTIAL OIL
   This oil is very strong, so it has to be used in little quantities. It helps to refresh, stimulate, and cool the skin due to its astringent properties which makes it ideal for acne prone skin but must be avoided in the first four months of pregnancy.
8. PATCHOULI ESSENTIAL OIL

It is amazing on cracked, chapped, acne, eczema, oily and matured skin. As it has a fungicidal, anti- microbial, astringent and deodorant function to the skin.

9. TEA TREE ESSENTIAL OIL

It is anti bacterial oil that will work great if blended with essential oils like lavender and peppermint. It is amazing on acne, oily, inflamed and rashes skin but applying too much of it can cause dryness to your skin, so it is advisable to add bit by bit until the right quantity is attained for each usage.

10. YLANG YLANG ESSENTIAL OIL

This oil is amazing for irritated, oily acne and general skin care, due to its strong scent; it is advisable to use few drops at a time until you get your desired aroma.

11. SANDALWOOD ESSENTIAL OIL

Very good for those with skin prone to acne, dry, cracked and chapped skin, amazing on wrinkles and mature skin.

12. SWEET ORANGE ESSENTIAL OIL

This oil is among the citrus essential oil that is not photo toxic but very effective on dull and oily skin.

CHAPTER SIX

NATURAL AND HOMEMADE WAY TO DO YOUR MAKE UP PRODUCTS

Many cosmetics we apply on our face, lips and around our eyes are embodied with harmful and deadly chemicals which are dangerous to our health, this is linked to cancer which can cause damage to our skin internally and externally.

These cosmetics, aside from being the carrier of cancer are also very expensive to use as you need a lot of money to afford them, so it is easy and cheap to make your own make up item and save your health and skin from being damage by chemicals from commercial products. Below are samples on how to do your make up products on your own at the comfort of you.

HOW TO MAKE YOUR BLUSHER OR BRONZER

Things needed are:
- Ground cinnamon   1 teaspoon (it is optional but it adds warmth and glow to your blusher)
- Arrow root powder or corn starch   ¼ cup
- Hibiscus powder   1 – 3 tablespoons

Put the arrow root or corn starch in a bowl and add the hibiscus powder slowly as you mix till you get your desired color then you add your cinnamon which is optional and mix well, pour into and old blusher can, it is ready for use.

HOMEMADE BLUSH

Things needed are:

- Arrow root powder or organic corn starch
- Beet root powder

Mix one part of arrow root powder to two parts of beet root powder if you need a bright pink color but if you need a darker color, swirl one part of arrow root powder to two parts of beet root powder and a little cocoa powder and pour into an old blush can, whenever you want to use, dip your blush brush into the can, tap off the excess powder and apply on the cheek bone.

CHAPTER SEVEN

HOW TO MAKE NATURAL FOUNDATION POWDER

Things needed are:

All the ingredients listed below depend on the color of your skin.

- Arrow root powder or corn starch (is a vital ingredient for any skin type, as it gives you a flawless look)
- Bentonite clay (it is optional but it has great advantage to your skin)
- Ginger (it is amazing for those with yellow pigments on their skin)
- French green clay or wheat grass powder (it is amazing for those with red pigments on their skin as green cancels red.
- Cocoa powder (darkens and add richness to the mixture, use a bit even though you are fair, but for dark colors, feel free to add more but be careful so it doesn't make you look darker)
- Bentonite clay (is optional but has great benefits for the skin)
- Cinnamon (darkens and add richness)

Add 1 tablespoon of arrow root powder or cornstarch to a bowl, depending on your skin color, and start mixing the rest ingredients in smaller quantity until you get your perfect match. To know whether the derived mixture matches your color or skin tone, dip your finger in the powder and rub is on the back of your hand, go outside to see if it blends, if it doesn't then you have to go and add more ingredients and try again. When you have arrived at the right color, use your brush to tap off any extra powder back into the jar and apply on your face in a circular motion just like any other loose powder foundation.

OR

- Cocoa powder
- Nutmeg
- Ground cinnamon
- Arrowroot powder
- Jojoba oil or olive oil or almond oil (optional)

Mix arrow root powder with cocoa powder, 1 teaspoon of arrow root powder for dark skin or 1 tablespoon for light skin, mix well and add cinnamon or nutmeg, mix until you reach your desired tone, add some jojoba or olive or almond oil to the mixture and press into an old compact. Use a brush when applying on the face.

HOW TO MAKE HEALING CONCEALER ON YOUR OWN.

Things needed are:

- Beeswax   0.8 teaspoon
- Magnesium stearate (optional, adds slip)   0.2 teaspoon
- Soluble titanium dioxide   1 ¼ teaspoon
- Sericite mica   ½ teaspoon
- Zeolite ultrafine clay   1 teaspoon
- Multani mitti clay   2 ¼ teaspoons
- Capuacu butter   1.4 or 1 ¼ teaspoons
- Cocoa butter   1 teaspoon
- Sea buck thorn seed oil (this fruit oil is likely to be so orange that it'll affect the color of the final product)   0.8 teaspoon
- Rosehip oil   0.8 teaspoon
- Vitamin E oil   0.2 teaspoon or 1 capsule
- Yellow iron oxide (use tiny measuring spoons for the oxides measurement)
- Red iron oxide
- Green chromium oxide

Melt beeswax, capuacu butter, cocoa butter, sea buckthorn seed oil, rosehip oil, vitamin E oil and magnesium stearate together in a small sauce pan over medium low heat, remove from heat and whisk in the titanium dioxide, sericite mica and clays, add 1 teaspoon of yellow iron oxide, 5/16 teaspoon of red and 3/16 teaspoon of brown, but if you like a red cancelling concealer, mix in a bit of green chromium oxide. Mix well; your concealer is ready for use.

CHAPTER EIGHT

HOW TO MAKE A CONCEALING COLOR CORRECTOR

Things needed are:

-	Sea buckthorn seed oil	0.4 or ¼ teaspoon
-	Jojoba oil	0.6 or 1/6 teaspoon
-	Vitamin oil	0.2 teaspoon or 1 capsule
-	Tamanu oil	0.4 or ¼ teaspoon
-	Cosmetic powder base	2 teaspoon
-	Yellow iron oxide	7/32 teaspoon
-	Brown iron oxide	a pinch
-	Red iron oxide	a pinch
-	Green chromium oxide	very very little

Put the cosmetic powder base in a coffee grinder and slowly start adding oxides, blending between additions and testing on your skin until more or less match your skin tone. Once it matches your skin tone, add minuscule bits of green oxide, testing the resultant powder out on a redder part of your skin so as to cancel red while doing all these, melt the oils in a small sauce pan over medium heat. Once you've got the powders right, mix 1 teaspoon of the melted oils with ½ teaspoon of the powders and mix together, or reheat in a micro wave for oils to melt well and mix to mash, as it mashes well pour into a shallow tin, do so till you finish mashing all the powders, apply to your face sparingly to avoid looking dead.

HOW TO MAKE MINERAL MAKE UP (LOOSE POWDER)

Things needed are:

-	magnesium stearate	1 teaspoon
-	sericite mica	1 tablespoon
-	zinc oxide	4 teaspoon
-	non micronized titanium dioxide	8 teaspoon
-	jojoba oil	¼ teaspoon
-	vitamin E oil	5 drops
-	yellow iron oxide	2 teaspoons
-	brown iron oxide	¼ teaspoon
-	red iron oxide	a pinch
-	rubbing alcohol (optional)	

Before starting this process, it is advisable to wear a dust mask to avoid inhaling the powder which might be dangerous to your health.

Mix the first four ingredients together, add half of the required measurements of the oxides, mash and grind all together using a mortar and pestle or press through a fine sieve or use both methods for best results, the more you mash and press out, the color of the oxides will come out, do not be hard on the oxides, once you have got your desired color, add Jojoba oil and vitamin E oil and mix with the powder then press through the fine sieve until all ingredients are well mixed. Your mineral make up is ready for use as a loose powder, you can also go further by adding a bit of rubbing alcohol to make a paste of the mixture, then you press it into an old powder compact pack, leave it open after putting it on the compact and let the alcohol evaporate off leaving you with a pressed powder.

OR

-	Pepper mint essential oil	20 drops
-	Cocoa powder	1 teaspoon
-	Arrow root powder	4 tablespoons

Mix the arrow root powder with the cocoa powder and see if the color suit your skin tone, if not add the ingredient bit by bit, dark colors require more cocoa powder while light skin tone requires more arrow root powder. When you reach your desired skin tone, add the pepper mint essential oil and pour it into a jar. Use a powder puff whenever you want to apply it on your face.

CHAPTER NINE

HOW TO MAKE SHEER OR SHIMMERING HIGHLIGHTING POWDER

This is used to brighten your face and face accenting.

Things needed are:

-	silver mica	¾ tablespoon
-	titanium dioxide	2 tablespoons
-	sericite mica	2 tablespoons
-	arrow root powder	1 tablespoon
-	silk powder	2 tablespoons
-	magnesium stearate	1 teaspoon
-	yellow iron oxide	1/32 teaspoon
-	red iron oxide	1/16 teaspoon
-	jojoba oil	8 drops

Put all the ingredients in a coffee grinder and blend very well, as you blend, stop at different intervals to scrape down the mixture on the walls of the grinder. When you finish blending, leave the lid on for some minutes so that the air or dust in the grinder settles to prevent the escape of the mixture to air, but with the presence of jojoba oil the mixture should not be too dusty. Turn the mixture into a shallow jar, your highlighting powder is ready to use, but if you want it to be shimmerier, add more silver mica.

HOW TO TURN YOUR LOOSE POWDER TO PRESSED POWDERS

In turning your loose powder to pressed powders, the major ingredient you need is magnesium stearate or zinc stearate as both are salts of stearic acid which helps to bind the powder together, and when you use magnesium stearate in larger quantities the creaminess it brings help to bind the powder together.

For 1 ¼ teaspoon or 9g of mineral make up.

Things needed are:

- magnesium stearate   1g or 0.2 teaspoon
- jojoba oil   25 drops
- used compressed powder pack
- coffee grinder

Firstly, you need to blend the mineral make up with the magnesium stearate in your coffee blender till it is uniform, then add jojoba oil but be careful not to add too much oil and blend but need to stop at intervals to scrape the particles on the wall of the grinder to it and continue until the powder looks granulate and chubby like a biscuit dough and starts to stick to the walls of the coffee blender, this shows that it has started pressing, all you need do is to pick up your used compressed powder pack and spread it evenly on it by laying a small piece of tissue or wax paper down over the makeup while you use a pressing tool to smooch the mixture down, add the mixture gently and slowly as you add more force to press it down, as you fill, take notice of the holes, thin spots and pay more attention to the corners and edges. When you have the entire make up in the compact, go over it again and make it as firm as you can, then you will have your loose powder turned to a well compressed powder.

CHAPTER TEN

HOW TO MAKE A MAKEUP REMOVER

1. OLIVE OIL PACK
   Things needed are:
   - vitamin E capsules   4
   - witch hazel or high proof vodka   ½ cup
   - olive oil   ½ cup

mix all the ingredients in a bowl and turn it into a jar and keep in your toiletry cabinet, shake well before use, due to lack of water in this mixture, it will last for 2 weeks before next preparation.

2. COCONUT OIL PACK

Things needed are:

   - Coconut oil   2 tablespoons
   - Baby wash or face wash   2 squirts
   - Warm water   4 cups
   - Lavender essential oil   12 drops
   - Frankincense essential oil   12 drops
   - Melaleuca essential oil   12 drops

Mix all the ingredients and pour into a squirt bottle, squirt into a cotton bud on each usage.

HOW TO MAKE NATURAL EYE LINER

Things needed are:

   - Distilled water or coconut oil   few drops
   - Activated charcoal   4 capsules

Put the activated charcoal in a container, add 2 drops of water or coconut oil and mix, continue to add the water or coconut oil and mix till the charcoal begins to clump. Pour the derived mixture into a shallow can and press down with your fingers until a smooth surface is achieved, whenever you want to use, dip your pointed brush into water before dipping it into the mixture and apply to your eyes.

HOMEMADE MASCARA

Things needed are:

- Activated charcoal   2 capsules
- Shea butter   1 teaspoon
- Coconut oil   ½ teaspoon
- Beeswax   1 ½ teaspoon
- Aloe vera gel   4 teaspoons
- Vitamin E oil   1 capsule

Melt coconut oil, shea butter, beeswax and aloe vera gel over boiling water, when it melts, add the activated charcoal and remove from heat. Stir and pour the mixture into a plastic bag, allow it to cool and open it at the tip so that you can transfer it easily into an old mascara tube. This mixture can last for maximum of 3 – 4 months since it contains natural ingredients.

CHAPTER ELEVEN

HOW TO MAKE LIP GLOSS

Things needed are:

- peppermint essential oil	20 drops
- vegetable glycerin	1 teaspoon
- vitamin E oil	2 capsules
- jojoba oil	3 teaspoons
- kukuinut oil	1 teaspoon
- beeswax	1 teaspoon
- virgin coconut oil	2 ½ teaspoons
- castor oil	6 ½ teaspoons
- micas for color	optional

Put the beeswax and other oils in a sauce pan and melt over a low heat or by placing it over a boiling water, when it melts, fill a shallow sauce pan with some ice cubes and place the sauce pan with the oils on it and whisk the oils till it is no longer liquid but soft and semi opaque, remove the pan from ice and add the vegetable glycerin and whisk zealously to dissolve the glycerin into the melted oils. Add essential oils to scent and micas if desired then pour the mixture into used lip gloss tubes with wand lid using a syringe.

LIP BALM

1. ALMOND OIL PACK

Things needed are:

-	Almond oil	1 tablespoon
-	Coconut oil	3 tablespoons
-	Cocoa butter	2 tablespoons
-	Grated beeswax	¼ cup

Put all the ingredients into a sauce pan to melt over low heat, stir and pour into a container, keep at room temperature.

2.   JOJOBA OIL PACK

-	Coconut oil	2 tablespoons
-	Cocoa butter	2 tablespoons
-	Beeswax	2 tablespoons
-	Jojoba oil	1 tablespoon
-	Vitamin E oil	1 teaspoon
-	Alkanent root powder or hibiscus powder (optional)	2 teaspoons
-	Essential oil of your choice	20 drops (optional)

Melt coconut oil, jojoba oil, cocoa butter and beeswax over a pot of boiling water, remove from heat, add vitamin E and the rest ingredients if using and pour into a jar, keep in a cool place.

CHAPTER TWELVE

HOW TO MAKE LIPSTICK USING HOMEMADE PRODUCTS

Lipsticks add beauty to our lips and makes us look attractive, but the usage of commercial lipsticks are very dangerous to our health as they contain chemicals which are harmful to our health and are the major cause of cancers due to the chemicals involve and these chemicals are easily absorb to the body system since it is apply in areas surrounding the mouth.

But if you do your own lipsticks using kitchen ingredients, it will be chemical free, cost free and skin friendly. Below are ways you can make your own chemical free lipsticks.

Things needed are:

- Coconut oil   1 teaspoon
- Shea butter or cocoa butter   1 teaspoon
- Beeswax   1 teaspoon
- Beet root powder   1/8 teaspoon or natural red food coloring for red color   1 drop
  For brown or tan color
- Organic cocoa powder   ¼ teaspoon
- Cinnamon or turmeric   a pinch(these two ingredients will replace the beet root powder or natural red food coloring if lipsticks with brown color)

Melt coconut oil, shea butter or cocoa butter, beeswax over boiling water, stir and remove from heat, add the rest ingredients and mix well. Decant into old lip sticks tubes.

RED ROSE LIPSTICK

Things needed are:

- cocoa butter   ¾ teaspoon

- shea butter	1 ½ teaspoon
- beeswax	¾ teaspoon
- avocado oil	2 teaspoons
- magnesium stearate	0.2 teaspoon
- peppermint essential oil	10 drops
- Australian red reef clay	2 teaspoons

Put the beeswax, shea butter, cocoa butter, avocado oil and magnesium stearate together in a sauce pan and place over a low heat or over boiling water, when it melts, remove from heat and add the clay and essential oil and stir well then pour into 4 lip balm tubes. Your lipstick is ready to be used.

CORAL LIPSTICK

Things needed are:

- Avocado oil	1 ¾ teaspoon
- Cocoa butter	¾ teaspoon
- Shea butter	1 ½ teaspoon
- Beewax	¾ teaspoon
- Magnesium stearate	0.2 teaspoon
- Peppermint essential oil	8 drops
- Red iron oxide	2 teaspoons
- Yellow iron oxide	¼ teaspoon
- Titanium oxide	1/8 teaspoon

When measuring the oxides, use a tiny measuring spoon.

Put the beeswax, shea butter, cocoa butter, avocado oil and magnesium stearate in a sauce pan and place over a low heat or over a boiling water to melt, but as it melts whisk the mixture well so that the magnesium stearate will melt along with the oils. Remove from heat, mix the oxides in another plate and add to the melt oils, stir and mash well with a spatula to combine all the ingredients together and add the essential oils and pour into 4 lip balm tubes.

CHAPTER THIRTEEN

HOW TO MAKE BABY BALM USING NATURAL INGREDIENTS

Things needed are:

- Castor oil   1 tablespoon
- Olive oil   2 tablespoons
- Shea butter   ¼ cup
- Cocoa butter   ¼ cup
- Essential oil of choice (frankincense, myrrh, chamomile and rose)   15 drops

Note that essential oils are to be use for children over 6 months.

Heat all ingredients except essential oil if using any over a pan of boiling water, stir until all ingredients melt and add essential oils, stir and pour into a jar for storage.

BABY BATH

1. MILK BATH

This needed are:

- Corn starch   ½ cup
- Dried milk   1 cup
- Lavender or chamomile essential oil   3 drops (optional)

Mix all the ingredients together in a jar for each usage. Milk is soothing and moisturizing to the skin as it gently cleanses the skin but if your child is allergic to cow milk, use goat milk as a substitute. Chamomile and lavender essential oils are naturally calming; this makes this bath perfect for fussy babies or toddlers. A small portion of the mixture is to be sprinkled in a warm bath on each usage. Note that essential oils are to be used for babies over 6 months of age.

2. FROTH BATH

Things needed are:

- Glycerin   1 teaspoon
- Water   1 cup
- Baby shampoo   3 tablespoons
- Essential oils   optional (10 drops) please use oil for babies who are 6 months or older.

Mix all these ingredients in a bowl and add to baby bath.

3. OAT MEAL BATH

All you need is a cup of oats, pour into your food processor and blend to fine powder. Sprinkle powder to your baby's bath before bathing your baby and see the amazing effects of this bath on your baby's skin.

CHAPTER FOURTEEN

HOW TO MAKE BABY BUM POWDER USING KITCHEN INGREDIENTS

Things needed are:

-	Cornstarch	¼ cup
-	White clay	1 tablespoon
-	Arrow root powder	¼ cup

Mix all ingredients together and use. Optionally you can add these essential oils.

-	Geranium	1 drop
-	Sweet orange	3 drops
-	Ylang ylang	2 drops

If you are using these essential oils, mix with the rest ingredients and store in a jar with sprinkle top, sprinkle moderately on your baby beddings or diaper area and avoid the face, if using on baby's body, shake powder into your hand away from baby and use to pat on him or her to avoid baby inhaling particles from the powder.

HOW TO MAKE BABY OIL USING KITCHEN INGREDIENTS

Things needed are:

-	Vitamin E capsules	3 drops
-	Grape seed or almond or sunflower oil	1 cup

Pierce the vitamin E capsules and squeeze the content into the base oil and shake well, pour into a used baby oil bottle and keep safe, to be used in bath as a lotion or massage oil.

Vegetable oils are more nourishing, moisturizing and soothing than mineral oils as it is amazing on cradle cap or eczema as it helps to loosen and heal it. It is very good natural massage oil.

Also, cradle cap can be sway away by rubbing a small amount of olive oil onto your baby's scalp, leave it on for 15 minutes and gently comb out the loose flakes with a soft baby brush then shampoo the hair and rinse.

CHAPTER FIFTEEN

DIAPER RASH CREAM

Diaper rash is a reaction on a baby's skin, which develops in the diaper covered region during the first three years of life; it is not a sign of parental neglect. It occurs mostly within the age range of 9 – 12 months of the baby's growing years, due to the fact that at this period, the baby mostly sits and eats solid foods which can change the acidity of the bowel movements. This reaction is often seen on babies no matter how careful their mothers are, but some precautions can be taken to prevent flare- ups. Rather than using commercial products which may make the rash get worse due to the chemicals used in the preparation of some diaper creams, it is advisable to use a homemade product which is chemical free and skin friendly as it does not involve the use of hash chemicals.

CAUSES OF DIAPER RASH

1. Body reaction: most at times your baby's skin may be allergic to some materials that touch their skin such as lotion, elastic in plastic pants, diapers or diaper wipes which may lead to reddish skin reactions on their skin.
2. Yeast infection: this happens commonly after the use of antibiotics, this infection is noticed in warm moist areas such as the mouth.
3. Irritation: the baby's skin gets reddish due to irritation caused by feaces, urine or cleaning agents, which affects the baby's skin from the wet diapers or acid in urine and this reaction is seen in areas where the diaper has rubbed.
4. Friction: this happens when the sensitive baby skin is rubbed by wet diapers, causing the area which the diaper has rubbed to be red and shiny. This is mostly the cause of most diaper rash infection in babies.

5. Diarrhea: this is when the movements of the bowels are loose and watery, due to this condition the baby's skin is expose to acid from the feaces which may cause rash on the baby's skin.

HOMEMADE DIAPER CREAMS

Zinc oxide powder is an ingredient needed most in the preparation of this cream but you may look at it as a hash chemical but it is not due to the following functions

- It helps to stimulate the immune system.
- It helps to protect your baby's skin by standing as a coat and barrier against wetness of your baby's skin.
- It consists of anti oxidant and anti bacterial properties which is amazing on your baby's sensitive skin.

1. COCONUT OIL PACK

Things needed are:

- Beeswax   one eighth of a cup
- Zinc oxide   three quarter of a teaspoon
- Coconut oil   two third of a cup

Melt the beeswax and coconut oil over a boiling water, when it melts, add the zinc oxide powder to the melted oils and stir to mix well using hand blender. Blend until the powder is well incorporated into the mixture to form a smooth paste without clumps. Pour it into a container and let it cool and solidify, it is ready to use, but for babies who are 6 months or older add essential oil like chamomile because of its calm effects.

2. COCOA BUTTER PACK

Things needed are:

- Zinc oxide   2 tablespoons
- Bentonite clay   3 tablespoons
- Cocoa butter   ¼ cup
- Coconut oil   ½ cup

- Beeswax	2 tablespoons
- Cod liver oil or olive oil	1 teaspoon
- Lanolin(optional)	1 teaspoon

Melt the beeswax, coconut oil; cod liver oil or olive oil, cocoa butter and lanolin (optional) in a sauce pan by placing it over a boiling water and stir as it melts. Pour it into a bowl and keep in the freezer to cool, when it cools remove and add zinc oxide and bentonite clay and stir for all the powders to mix well with the oils then return the mixture into the freezer for 10 minutes for the mixture to solidify. Remove from the freezer and whip with a hand blender until it stiffs , return to the freezer for another 5 minutes and whip thereafter until a thick lotion texture is seen then pour into a jar and keep in a cool place, but if the mixture is not firming up as you blend, return to the freezer and blend later. This mixture has a life span of over 6 months.

CHAPTER SIXTEEN

BREAST FIRMING

Breast sagging is a natural process in women as it happens according to your age when your breast lose its suppleness and elasticity. The breast do not have muscles rather they are have connective tissues and milk It happens mostly when a woman reaches age 40 and above. This process can occur earlier than expected due to some factors, such as breast feeding, pregnancy, menopause, and increase or lose weight, doing strenuous exercise, nutritional deficiencies and wearing a poorly fitting bra. Also, some diseases or illnesses can cause your breast to sag such as: cancer or respiratory conditions like tuberculosis, consuming excess nicotine, alcohol; and carbonated beverages factors that causes breast sagging.

Breasts do not have muscles, they are made up of fats, connective tissues and milk producing glands, to make them firm and in good shape, they need proper care to make them look attractive to our loved ones. Below are various ways you can put your breasts back to shape and look attractive. After the application of each method, endeavor to put on a fitted bra or pull up bra for best results.

1. OLIVE OIL
   Olive oil has high anti oxidants and fatty acids content that are able to restore the damage caused by free radicals which cause the breast to sag. Also they will help to improve your skin tone and textures; it enhances skin tightness, making it look attractive and flawless. It can be used in the following ways to restore or prevent breast sagging.

Apply some olive oil to your palms, rub together to generate heat and rub it on your breast in an upward motion for 15 minutes, this action will help to increase blood flow and help repair damaged cells in the breast. Do this 5 times a week for best results. Also you can use jojoba oil or avocado oil or argan oil to perform this process.

2. CUCUMBER PACK

Cucumber helps to tone the skin naturally, it combination with egg yolk helps to treat sagging breast because egg yolk has high level of protein and vitamins. All you need to do is to puree 1 cucumber in a blender, mix 1 egg yolk and 1 teaspoon of butter and mix to form a paste. Apply this mixture to your breast for 30 minutes and wash off thereafter, do this once a week for best results as it will help to strengthen your breast tissues.

3. FENUGREEK PACK

Fenugreek contains vitamins and anti oxidants which fights against free radicals damage which the main cause of breast are sagging, it helps to tighten, lift and smoothen the skin around the breasts leaving your breast firm and attractive.

All you need to do is to mix ¼ cup of fenugreek powder with enough water to form a thick paste. Use this paste to massage your breasts and leave it on for 10 minutes before washing off with warm water, do this twice a week for best results.

4. ICE PACK

Take 2 ice cubes and massage them on your breasts for 1 minutes (please do not go beyond a minute to prevent numbness), dry your breasts and put on a fitting bra immediately then sit or lie in a reclining position for 30 minutes. This can be done several times a day for best results.

5. EGG WHITE PACK

Egg white is amazing in the treatment of sagging breasts as it contains astringents and some skin nourishing properties such as hydro lipid which helps to lift loose skin around the breasts area. You can apply it in two ways which are as follows:

❖ Whisk 1 egg white until you get the foamy texture, apply this to your breasts and leave on for 30 minutes before washing off with cucumber or onion juice and later cold water.

❖ Whisk 1 egg white with 1 tablespoon of plain yogurt and honey each, apply this mixture to your breasts and leave on for 20 minutes before rinsing off with cold water. Do this once a week for best results.

6. SWIMMING

This also helps to tighten up the muscles responsible for holding up the breasts. It is advisable for those with sagging breasts to engage in swimming exercise so as to lift their drooping breasts.

CHAPTER SEVENTEEN

HOW TO LIGHTEN DARK SKIN AROUND YOUR PUBIC AREA USING KITCHEN INGREDIENTS.

Discolorations between the thighs and pubic area is a cosmetic issue which causes embarrassment to major women who intend to put on bikinis, shorts and miniskirts, but due to this such clothing turns out to be a major turn off. Fortunately, this issue is not a medical issue because it happens due to many reasons and mistakes we do with clothes we put on.

   Hyper pigmentation of the bikini line or pubic area is commonly caused by genetic factors and some people tend to develop excess pigmentation in their pubic area than others due to the following reasons:

1. Over exposure to harmful ultra violet sunrays.
2. Excessive sweating.
3. Wearing polyester under wear.
4. Regular shaving.
5. Constant friction between thighs due to wearing clothes that is too tight.
6. Being affected with some kind of disease.
7. Accumulation of dead skin.

The pubic area as we all know is a very delicate area where we cannot use commercial products such as bleaching creams or skin whitening products to lighten it, rather it is advisable to use kitchen ingredients to get rid of the embarrassing dark skin and when applying these ingredients, you need to wait patiently for results. The methods involved are listed below:

1. LEMON JUICE PACK

This method helps you to get rid of dead skin and tone your skin evenly. It also helps to regenerate healthy skin cells leaving your pubic area light and healthy. This method can be done in two ways, which are as follows:

- ➤ Get a lemon and cut it into half, use each to rub your pubic area gently and leave on for 15 minutes before washing off with warm water.
- ➤ Mix lemon juice with 1 tablespoon of plain yogurt and ½ teaspoon of honey, apply this mixture to your bikini line and wash off after 10 minutes of application with cool water and apply a moisturizer or coconut oil to your skin after washing as lemon juice dries out your skin.

2. CUCUMBER JUICE PACK

This method helps to eliminates skin darkness as it controls your skin production of melanin which is the main cause of dark skin; it also keeps the skin hydrated and glowing due to its high water content. This method can be applied in two ways which are:

- ✓ Mixing 2 tablespoons of cucumber juice to ½ tablespoons each of lemon juice and turmeric powder and apply the mixture to your bikini area, wash off after 10 minutes of application with cool water. Do this once a week for best results.
- ✓ Get a cucumber, extract the juice and apply it all over the delicate area and leave it on for 15 minutes before washing off with cool water. Do this twice a week for best results.

3. ALOE VERA PACK

This helps to restore skin cells and encourage the regeneration of new healthy ones naturally. All you need to do is to get an aloe vera leaf, extract the gel and apply it directly to the sensitive area. Wash off 20 minutes after application, for best results do it once daily.

4. TOMATOES PACK

This method helps to get rid of dead skin from the pubic area due to the fact that tomatoes are natural bleaching agents. All you need to do is to get a tomato, puree it and apply to the delicate area, wash off after 10 minutes of application with cool water. Do this once daily for best results.

5. ALMOND PACK

This method helps to lighten the pubic area, and encourages even skin tone. This can be achieved in two ways which are:

- ❖ Get 6 whole almonds and soak it overnight, the next morning, grind them into a smooth paste and mix 1 tablespoons of milk to it, apply this mixture to your pubic area for 15 minutes before washing off the paste gently in circular motions. Do this thrice weekly for best results.
- ❖ Warm 2 tablespoons of almond oil and use it to massage the pubic area for 5 minutes before going to bed at night.

6. ORANGE PEEL PACK

This method helps to lighten dark blotches and eliminate them in no time, this can be done by gathering orange peels, sun dry them, grind them into fine paste. Mix 1 tablespoon of orange peel powder to 2 tablespoons of plain yogurt and 1 teaspoon of honey, apply this mixture to your bikini line and allow it to dry. Scrub off the paste with wet hands and rinse later with cool water. Do this twice a week for best results.

7. PAPAYA PACK

This method works wonders in lightening the pubic area fast, all you need to do is to rub ¼ cup of papaya pulp on the dark area of your bikini line for 5 minutes and wash off after 15 minutes of application with cool water. Do this every day for best results.

8. BAKING SODA PACK

This method is only meant for those who do not have sensitive skin as it may cause some irritation, but it helps to prevent excess sweating in the pubic area which is the major cause of skin discolorations and skin folds on the pubic area. All you need to do is to mix baking soda with a little water to form a paste and apply this mixture to the pubic area, allow it to dry before rinsing off with cool water. Do this twice a week for best results.

9. MILK

This method helps to eliminate skin pigmentation and lighten the skin in the process; this can be carried out in this form:

Pour a cup of cold milk to a bowl and dip a cotton cloth into it, place this cloth on the dark areas of the pubic area for 5 minutes, do this continuously for some times before massaging the area for some minutes and rinse off with water. Do this twice daily for best results.

CHAPTER EIGHTEEN

ARMPIT CLEANSING

Armpit cleansing is good for everyone but necessary for those who have been wearing conventional anti per spirants or deodorants for quite some times now. Armpit cleansing will not only clean out build up toxins on the skin but will reduce the amount and odor of sweat from the body, it also boost the body immune system and reduce the risks of having cancer.

Sweating is very healthy because it helps to cool the body system, eliminates toxins and encourages proper immune function; this makes some people to avoid the use of anti perspirant.

REASONS WHY YOU NEED AN ARMPIT CLEANSING

1. Those who experience an uncomfortable rash or excessive sweating, and also their armpits produce an offensive smell due to the use of several deodorants. This is due to the over production of bad bacteria aggravated to worse odors when you stop using these deodorants. But with a good armpit cleanse, you will put those bacteria to check and smell naturally good and fresh every day.
2. We all have a sticky or filmy build up in our armpits which do not wash away even after shower. This is as a result of the active ingredients known as aluminum which clogs the pores to stop sweating; this ingredient is mostly found in some deodorants. But with an armpit cleanse, you can get rid of some of these chemicals in the skin tissues surrounding the armpit easily.
3. If you are someone who gets sick or notice enlarged lymph nodes on the neck or in your armpit, this is due to the fact that your lymphatic system is struggling to release chemicals and other foreign invaders out of your system. Which causes a sluggish immune system, then you need an armpit cleanse to put this to check.

RESULTS OF A GOOD ARMPIT CLEANSE

When you have an armpit cleanse, you will notice the following:

- Reduced or less odor emanating from your armpit even without wearing a natural deodorant.
- Reduced irritation and perspiration after using natural deodorants.
- No more products build up in your armpit.
- A well improved lymphatic function and illness free body system.

To support your armpit healths reduce the intake of the following:

- Caffeine.
- Alcohol.
- Garlic and onions.
- Processed fatty and sugary foods.
- Spicy foods.

For a healthy armpit, use only natural deodorant and never try your hands on conventional chemical- laden anti perspirants or deodorants. This is a sample of a natural deodorant:

Things needed are:

| - | Bentonite clay | 1 tablespoon |
| - | Raw apple cider vinegar | 1 teaspoon |

Mix these two ingredients together with two spoons of water to form a paste and apply the mixture to your armpit, leave it on for 15 minutes before shower.

CHAPTER NINETEEN

DEODORANT

Deodorants contain dangerous unpronounceable ingredients or chemicals which tend to be very dangerous to our health. It contains a class of substance called **paraben** which helps to stop the growth of bacteria, mold and yeast but in turns have a negative effect on the body's endocrine system. It also contains a chemical called **carcinogen** which blocks the sweat ducts and encourages the growth of breast cancer cells. Some even contains pesticides which are used in form of anti bacteria agent called **triclosan** which is commonly found in most deodorants, soaps and personal care products. This chemical disturbs the regulation of hormones in the body and stimulates antibiotic resistance bacteria which tend to be very dangerous to human health.

  Furthermore, your skin can react badly to deodorants which may result to itchiness, rash, swelling or redness due to the presence of these chemicals. Aside from being dangerous to human's health, it tends to be very expensive to afford and causes the formation of tough stains on our clothes. Below are ways to make natural deodorant using kitchen ingredients which are skin and environment friendly, easy and cheap to produce.

1. SHEA BUTTER PACK
   Things needed are:
   - Baking soda   3 tablespoons
   - Coconut oil   3 tablespoons
   - Shea butter   2 tablespoons
   - Arrow root or organic corn starch   2 tablespoons (optional)
   - Essential oils (optional)

Melt shea butter and coconut oil over boiling water, remove from heat, add baking soda and arrow root (if using) but if not using add more arrow root , add essential oil (if using), pour the mixture into a jar on pour into an old deodorant stick for easier use.

2. COCONUT OIL DEODORANT

Things needed are:

- Arrow root powder or organic corn starch   ¼ cup
- Coconut oil   6 tablespoons
- Baking soda   ¼ cup
- Essential oil (optional)

Mix the baking powder and arrow root powder together, mash the solid coconut oil into the mixture and mix well, add essential oils if you which and pour into an old deodorant container for easy use. But if your body reacts to coconut oil, use almond, jojoba or avocado oil. If your body also reacts to baking soda, use diluted lemon juice or apple cider vinegar alone or with essential oils.

HOW TO MAKE A SPRAY DEODORANT

Things needed are:

- Magnesium oil   4 tablespoons
- Essential oil (optional)   10 or 15 drops

Pour magnesium oil into a glass spray bottle, add essential oils (if using), whenever you want to use, spray a small amount of this mixture under your arms and rub gently for 5 seconds to dry off.

BAKING SODA DEODORANT

Things needed are:

- Arrow root powder or cornstarch (arrow root is preferred)   ¼ cup
- Baking soda   ¼ cup
- Coconut oil   8 tablespoons

Mix baking soda and arrow root powder/ cornstarch together and slowing add the coconut oil, mix with a spoon or hand blender until it is firm but pliable texture but if the mixture is too wet, add more arrow root powder or cornstarch until it thickens, then scoop it into an old deodorant dispenser or a container and apply with your fingers with each use.